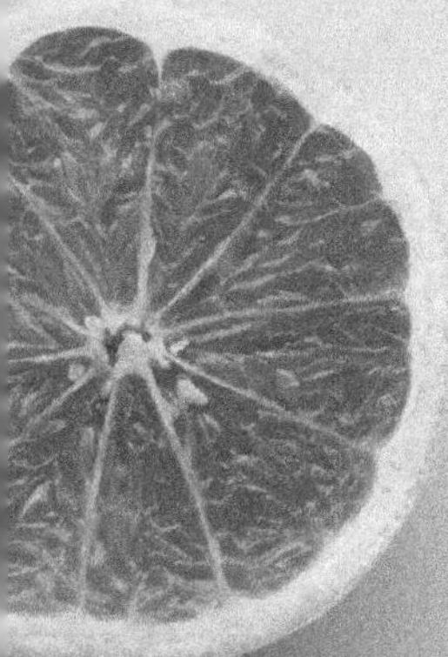

In My Gut Feelings

The guide to a healthier gut in 5 months naturally

Maryonique Elmore

Chapter Outline

Chapter 1: Introduction to Gut Health
- Importance of gut health for overall well-being
- How gut health affects children and mothers
- Overview of the microbiome and its role

Chapter 2: Understanding Common Gut Health Issues
- Common gut health issues in mothers and children
- Symptoms to watch out for
- Impact of diet on gut health

Chapter 3: Foundations of a Healthy Gut-Friendly Diet
- Basics of a gut-friendly diet
- Importance of fiber, prebiotics, and probiotics
- Foods to avoid for gut health

Chapter 4: Planning Balanced Meals for the Family
- How to plan meals that support gut health
- Balancing macronutrients for optimal digestion
- Meal prepping tips for busy mothers

Chapter 5: Breakfast Ideas for Gut Health
- Nutritious and quick breakfast options
- Meal ideas for gut-friendly smoothies and overnight oats
- Importance of starting the day with fiber and hydration

Chapter 6: Lunch and Dinner Meal Ideas
- Easy-to-make lunch and dinner Meal Ideas
- Incorporating a variety of vegetables and whole grains
- One-pot meals and batch cooking strategies

Chapter 7: Snack Ideas to Support Gut Health
- Healthy snack options for mothers and kids
- Importance of snacks in maintaining energy
- Homemade snacks versus store-bought options

Chapter 8: Desserts and Treats Without Compromising Gut Health
- Healthier dessert alternatives
- Meal ideas for gut-friendly sweets and treats
- Moderation and balance in indulgence

Chapter 9: Special Considerations: Gut Health During Pregnancy and Breastfeeding
- Nutritional needs during pregnancy and lactation
- Foods to support gut health during these stages
- Tips for managing digestive discomfort

Chapter 10: Lifestyle Tips for Sustaining Gut Health
- Beyond diet: Importance of sleep and stress management
- Incorporating exercise for overall health
- Long-term strategies for maintaining gut health

Each chapter will expand into detailed sections with tips, meal ideas, meal plans, and actionable advice tailored to mothers looking to improve their own gut health and that of their families.

Chapter 1: The importance of Gut Health

Good gut health is essential for overall well-being as it impacts digestion, immune function, and mental health. For mothers juggling childcare, daily responsibilities, and in some cases work, optimizing gut health can significantly improve their vitality and well-being."

The Importance of Gut Health

The microbiome is an ecosystem of trillions of bacteria, fungi, and other microorganisms that primarily reside in our digestive tract. It plays a crucial role in breaking down food and synthesizing vitamins, and regulating our immune system. Research has connected the health of our gut microbiome to various aspects of our well-being, including the risk of chronic diseases like obesity, diabetes, and autoimmune conditions.

Having a healthy gut is important for both mothers and their children. It helps with digestion and absorbing nutrients, which is crucial for the well-being of mothers and the development of their children's microbiomes. The microbial environment during the infant stage and early childhood stage is essential for the development of the immune system and long-term health outcomes.

Factors Affecting Gut Health

There are several factors that can influence the balance of our gut microbiota, including diet, lifestyle, stress levels, medications, and environmental exposures. A diet that is rich in fiber, fruits, vegetables, and fermented foods promotes diversity within the microbiome and supports the growth of beneficial bacteria that contribute to gut health. For mothers who breastfeed, it is vital after pregnancy for improving gut health. On the other hand, diets high in processed foods, sugars, and artificial additives can disrupt this balance, potentially leading to inflammation, digestive issues, and a weakened immune response.

The Bottom Line

Gut health is crucial for everyone, but it holds particular importance for women due to several reasons:

1. **Digestive Health:** A healthy gut ensures proper digestion and absorption of nutrients, which is essential for overall well-being and energy levels. Women often have specific nutritional needs, especially during pregnancy and breastfeeding, making optimal digestion vital.

2. **Immune Function:** A significant portion of the immune system resides in the gut. A healthy gut microbiome helps defend against pathogens and supports immune responses, which is crucial for women's health throughout their lives.

3. **Hormonal Balance:** The gut microbiota plays a role in metabolizing hormones, including estrogen. Imbalances in gut bacteria can potentially lead to hormonal disturbances, affecting menstrual cycles, fertility, and menopausal symptoms.

Mental Health: The gut-brain axis connects the gut and the brain through neural, hormonal, and immune pathways. A healthy gut contributes to better mental health outcomes, reducing the risk of anxiety and depression, which disproportionately affect women.

The bottom line

5. **Weight Management:** The composition of gut bacteria influences metabolism and how energy from food is stored. Maintaining a healthy gut can support healthy weight management, which is often a concern for women.

6. **Inflammatory Conditions:** Gut health is closely linked to inflammation levels in the body. Chronic inflammation is associated with various diseases, including autoimmune conditions like rheumatoid arthritis, which are more prevalent in women.

7. **Overall Longevity and Quality of Life:** A healthy gut contributes to longevity and overall quality of life by reducing the risk of chronic diseases and supporting optimal bodily functions.

Many mothers may experience common gut-related issues such as bloating, constipation, or food intolerance, which can impact their daily lives and overall well-being. Recognizing the symptoms and understanding the underlying causes can empower mothers to make informed dietary and lifestyle choices that support optimal gut health.

Conclusion

In conclusion, Chapter 1 serves as a foundational introduction to the critical role of gut health in maternal and child well-being. By understanding the importance of maintaining a healthy gut microbiome and recognizing factors that influence gut health, mothers can embark on a journey towards improved vitality, enhanced immune function, and overall better health outcomes for themselves and your children.

Chapter 2: Understanding the Gut Microbiome

This chapter delves into the intricate world of the gut microbiome, shedding light on its composition, functions, and the factors influencing its balance.

What is the Gut Microbiome?

Think of your gut as a thriving community that houses trillions of bacteria, viruses, fungi, and other microorganisms. This community, known as the gut microbiome, creates a complex ecosystem that is unique to each person. The microbiome is not just a passive entity; it actively communicates with our body, affecting everything from digestion and metabolism to immune function and mood.

Factors that Influence Gut Health

Several factors impact the delicate balance of the gut microbiome:

Diet

The foods we eat directly influence the composition of our gut microbiota. A diet rich in fiber from fruits, vegetables, and whole grains promotes the growth of beneficial bacteria, while excessive sugar and processed foods can disrupt this balance.

Lifestyle Choices

Exercise, sleep patterns, and stress levels also affect gut health. Regular physical activity and adequate sleep contribute positively however chronic stress can alter gut microbiota composition and function.

Medications

Antibiotics, while essential for fighting infections, can inadvertently disrupt the gut microbiome by killing off harmful and beneficial bacteria. Other medications, such as proton pump inhibitors and non-steroidal anti-inflammatory drugs, may also impact gut health.Antibiotics, while crucial for combating infections, can disturb the gut microbiome by killing off both harmful and beneficial bacteria. Other medications, such as nonsteroidal anti-inflammatory drugs, may also have an impact on gut health.

Factors that Influence Gut Health

Environment

Environmental factors, such as exposure to pollutants and certain chemicals, can influence the diversity and resilience of the gut microbiome.

Impact of Gut Health on Mothers

During pregnancy, changes in the microbiome occur naturally to support the mother and baby's health. Beyond reproduction, mothers often juggle multiple responsibilities, which can lead to stress and irregular eating habits. These factors can affect gut health while impacting overall well-being and immunity. By understanding how to support a healthy gut, mothers can enhance their resilience to stress, boost their energy levels, and maintain optimal health.

Factors that Influence Gut Health

Why Gut Health Matters

The gut microbiome is not only essential for digestion but also acts as a guardian of our immune system. Approximately 70% of our immune cells reside in the gut, interacting with the microbiome to regulate immune responses and protect against infections. A diverse and balanced microbiome contributes to better immune function, reducing the risk of allergies, autoimmune diseases, and gastrointestinal disorders.

Conclusion

By prioritizing a diet rich in fiber, embracing stress-management techniques, and maintaining a healthy lifestyle, mothers can cultivate a thriving gut microbiome that enhances vitality and resilience. In the following chapters, we will explore practical strategies and delicious meal ideas designed to nourish both the body and microbiome, fostering long-lasting health benefits for mothers and their families.

Chapter 3: Key Nutrients for Gut Health

A healthy gut thrives on a balanced diet rich in key nutrients. In this chapter, we will explore the essential nutrients crucial for nurturing gut health, understanding their roles, and identifying sources that can easily be incorporated into daily meals.

Fiber: Nature's Gut Health Hero

Fiber is a non-digestible carbohydrate found in plant-based foods like fruits, vegetables, whole grains, nuts, and seeds. It serves as the primary food source for beneficial gut bacteria, known as probiotics, helping them flourish and maintain a healthy balance within the gut microbiome. There are two main types of fiber: soluble and insoluble.

Key Nutrients for Gut Health

Soluble Fiber

This type of fiber dissolves in water to form a gel-like substance in the digestive tract. It helps regulate blood sugar levels and cholesterol, while also promoting the growth of beneficial bacteria. Good sources include oats, legumes (beans and lentils), apples, and citrus fruits.

Insoluble Fiber

Unlike soluble fiber, insoluble fiber does not dissolve in water and adds bulk to stool, promoting regular bowel movements and preventing constipation. Whole grains (such as wheat, brown rice, and quinoa), vegetables (like broccoli, carrots, and spinach), and nuts/seeds (like almonds and flaxseeds) are rich sources of insoluble fiber.

Key Nutrients for Gut Health

Prebiotics vs. Probiotics: Nurturing Your Gut

While probiotics are live microorganisms found in fermented foods like yogurt, kefir, sauerkraut, and kimchi, prebiotics are indigestible fibers that serve as food for these beneficial bacteria. By consuming both prebiotics and probiotics, mothers can optimize their gut health by promoting the growth of beneficial bacteria and maintaining a healthy balance in the microbiome.

Probiotics

These live microorganisms can help restore and maintain a healthy balance of gut bacteria, supporting digestion and immunity. Yogurt with live cultures, kombucha, miso, and fermented vegetables are excellent sources of probiotics.

Prebiotics

Found in foods rich in fiber, prebiotics promote the growth of beneficial bacteria in the gut. Incorporating foods like onions, garlic, bananas, asparagus, and chicory root into the diet can help nourish these microbes.

Key Nutrients for Gut Health

Essential Vitamins and Minerals

Several vitamins and minerals play crucial roles in supporting gut health and overall well-being:

Vitamin D

Besides its well-known role in bone health, vitamin D helps regulate the immune system and may influence gut microbiota composition. Fatty fish (like salmon and mackerel), egg yolks, and fortified dairy products are good dietary sources.

B Vitamins

These water-soluble vitamins, including B6, B12, and folate, are needed for energy metabolism and nerve function. Whole grains, leafy greens, legumes, and animal products are excellent sources.

Key Nutrients for Gut Health

Magnesium

This mineral supports muscle and nerve function, energy production, and bone strength. Nuts, seeds, whole grains, and leafy green vegetables are rich sources of magnesium.

Zinc

Essential for immune function, wound healing, and protein synthesis, zinc which is found in lean meats, shellfish, legumes, seeds, and dairy products.

Nutrient-Rich Foods into Your Diet

To optimize gut health, include a variety of nutrient-dense foods in your daily meals and snacks. Incorporating colorful fruits and vegetables, whole grains, lean proteins, nuts, seeds, and fermented foods can provide a broad spectrum of vitamins, minerals, fiber, and beneficial bacteria essential for supporting a healthy gut.

Key Nutrients for Gut Health

Conclusion

By understanding the importance of fiber, prebiotics, probiotics, and essential nutrients, mothers can take proactive steps toward supporting their gut health and overall well-being. In the upcoming chapters, we will explore useful meal-planning strategies and delicious meal ideas designed to nourish the gut, making it easier for mothers to prioritize their health and the health of their families.

Chapter 4: Meal Planning Basics

Meal planning is a powerful tool that mothers can prioritize healthy eating amidst busy schedules. In this chapter, we'll explore the fundamentals of meal planning, offering practical tips to streamline grocery shopping, optimize kitchen efficiency, and prepare nutritious meals that support gut health.

The Importance of Meal Planning

For mothers juggling multiple responsibilities, meal planning provides structure and efficiency in the kitchen. By planning meals ahead, mothers can ensure their families consume balanced and nutritious meals throughout the week. This proactive approach not only saves time but also reduces stress associated with last-minute meal decisions.

Meal Planning Basics

Tips for Effective Meal Planning

1. Set Aside Dedicated Planning Time: Choose a specific day each week to plan your meals. This could involve browsing recipes, creating a shopping list, setting a timer to schedule meal planning and organizing your weekly menu.

2. Consider Your Family's Preferences and Dietary Needs: Take into account any dietary restrictions, allergies, or preferences when selecting recipes. This ensures that everyone in the family enjoys the meals while meeting their nutritional needs.

3. Create a Weekly Menu: Plan breakfasts, lunches, dinners, and snacks for the upcoming week. Variety is key to a balanced diet, so aim for a mix of proteins, vegetables, whole grains, and fruits.

Meal Planning Basics

Tips for Effective Meal Planning

4. Make a Detailed Shopping List: Once your menu is planned, create a shopping list. Organize your list by food categories (produce, dairy, pantry items) to streamline your grocery shopping experience.

5. Batch Cooking and Meal Prep: Prepare ingredients in advance to streamline cooking during busy weekdays.

6. Use Leftovers Creatively: Plan meals that can yield leftovers for quick lunches or dinners.

Meal Planning Basics

Smart Grocery Shopping Strategies

1. Stick to Your List: Avoid impulse purchases by sticking to your pre-planned shopping list. This will help you avoid unnecessary items and stay within your budget.

2. Shop Seasonally and Locally: Choose seasonal produce when possible, as it tends to be fresher and more affordable. Consider visiting local farmers' markets for fresh, locally sourced ingredients.

3. Read Labels Mindfully: When purchasing packaged foods, read labels carefully to identify hidden sugars, unhealthy fats, and artificial additives.

Meal Planning Basics

Organizing Your Kitchen for Efficiency

1. Keep Essentials Accessible: Organize your kitchen pantry and refrigerator to keep essentials like grains, canned goods, spices, and condiments easily accessible.

2. Invest in Storage Containers: Use a variety of storage containers to keep prepped ingredients and leftovers organized. Clear containers allow you to see what's inside and prevent food waste.

3. Kitchen Tools and Gadgets: Invest in essential kitchen tools like sharp knives, cutting boards, measuring cups, and a blender or food processor to streamline meal preparation.

Meal Planning Basics

Organizing Your Kitchen for Efficiency

Conclusion

Embracing meal planning as a fundamental aspect of healthy eating enables mothers to effortlessly integrate nutritious meals into their family's daily routine. With careful planning, efficient shopping, and organized meal preparation, mothers can prioritize their own health and well-being while nourishing their families with delicious, gut-friendly meals. In the upcoming chapters, we will explore specific meal ideas and recipe ideas tailored to support gut health and promote overall vitality for mothers and their loved ones health and well-being while nurturing their families with delicious, gut-friendly meals.

Chapter 5: Building a Gut-Healthy Plate

Creating balanced meals that support gut health is essential for mothers looking to optimize their overall well-being and that of their families. In this chapter, we'll explore the principles of building a gut-healthy plate, emphasizing nutrient-rich foods that nourish the gut microbiome and promote digestive health.

Building a Gut-Healthy Plate

Components of a Gut-Healthy Plate

A gut-healthy plate consists of a balance of macronutrients (carbohydrates, proteins, fats) and includes a variety of colorful fruits, vegetables, whole grains, lean proteins, and healthy fats. Here's how to build a nutritious plate that supports gut health:

1. Fill Half Your Plate with Vegetables and Fruits: Vegetables and fruits are rich in fiber, vitamins, minerals, and antioxidants that support gut health. Aim for a colorful variety, including leafy greens, cruciferous vegetables (like broccoli and cauliflower), berries, citrus fruits, and more.

2. Choose Whole Grains: Whole grains such as brown rice, quinoa, oats, and whole wheat provide fiber, B vitamins, and essential minerals. These nutrients promote digestive regularity and support a diverse gut microbiome.

Building a Gut-Healthy Plate

Components of a Gut-Healthy Plate

3. Incorporate Lean Proteins: Include lean proteins like poultry, fish, beans, lentils, tofu, and lean cuts of beef or pork. Protein is essential for muscle repair and maintenance, and certain amino acids from protein sources also contribute to a healthy gut lining.

4. Include Healthy Fats: Healthy fats found in nuts, seeds, avocados, and olive oil provide essential fatty acids that support gut health and reduce inflammation. Omega-3 fatty acids are beneficial for gut lining integrity and overall health.

Building a Gut-Healthy Plate

Components of a Gut-Healthy Plate

5. Add Fermented Foods: Fermented foods like yogurt with live cultures, kefir, kimchi, and kombucha which contains probiotics that introduce beneficial bacteria into the gut. Regular consumption of these foods can enhance gut diversity and function.

Portion Control and Mindful Eating

Beyond selecting nutrient-rich foods, practicing portion control and mindful eating habits is key to supporting gut health:

Listen to Your Hunger Cues: Eat slowly and pay attention to your body's hunger and fullness signals. Avoid overeating and aim for balanced portions that satisfy your nutritional needs without excess.

Building a Gut-Healthy Plate

Portion Control and Mindful Eating

Stay Hydrated: Drink plenty of water throughout the day and limit sugary beverages that can negatively impact gut health.

Gut-Healthy Meals

Here are examples of meals that embody the principles of a gut-healthy plate:

Breakfast: Greek yogurt topped with berries and a sprinkle of chia seeds, paired with whole grain toast spread with almond butter.

Lunch: Quinoa salad with mixed greens, cherry tomatoes, cucumber, avocado, and grilled chicken, drizzled with a lemon-tahini dressing.

Dinner: Baked salmon served with roasted sweet potatoes and steamed broccoli, seasoned with olive oil and herbs.

Building a Gut-Healthy Plate

Creating Balanced Snacks

Snacks can also contribute to gut health when chosen wisely:

Fresh Fruit with Nuts: Apple slices paired with almonds or walnuts provide fiber, vitamins, minerals, and healthy fats.

Vegetable Sticks with Hummus: Carrot and celery sticks dipped in hummus offer fiber, protein, and beneficial nutrients.

Building a Gut-Healthy Plate

Conclusion

By building meals around nutrient-dense foods that support gut health, mothers can nourish themselves and their families with delicious and wholesome meals. Adopting these principles of a gut-healthy plate not only supports digestive health but also contributes to overall vitality and well-being.

Chapter 6: Gut-Healthy Breakfast Ideas

Breakfast sets the tone for the day, providing essential nutrients and energy to kickstart metabolism and support overall well-being. For mothers seeking to prioritize gut health, choosing nutrient-dense breakfast options is key. This chapter explores gut-healthy breakfast ideas that are easy to prepare, delicious, and packed with ingredients that support a thriving gut microbiome.

Gut-Healthy Breakfast Ideas

The Importance of a Gut-Healthy Breakfast

Starting the day with a balanced breakfast that includes fiber, probiotics, and essential nutrients sets a positive foundation for gut health. A nutrient-rich breakfast not only supports digestion but also fuels energy levels, enhances mental clarity, and promotes overall vitality throughout the day.

Gut-Healthy Breakfast Components

When planning a gut-healthy breakfast, consider incorporating the following components:

Gut-Healthy Breakfast Ideas

Gut-Healthy Breakfast Components

1. Fiber-Rich Foods: Fiber supports digestive regularity and feeds beneficial gut bacteria like whole grains, fruits, vegetables, nuts, and seeds to increase fiber intake.

2. Probiotic Foods: Include probiotic-rich foods like yogurt with live cultures, kefir, or fermented vegetables.

3. Healthy Fats: Incorporate sources of healthy fats such as avocado, nuts, seeds, and olive oil.

Gut-Healthy Breakfast Ideas

Gut-Healthy Breakfast Ideas

1. Overnight Oats with Berries and Greek Yogurt:
- Combine rolled oats, chia seeds, and milk (or yogurt) in a jar overnight.
- In the morning, top with fresh berries, a dollop of Greek yogurt, and a sprinkle of nuts or seeds for added crunch and healthy fats.

2. Smoothie Bowl with Greens and Probiotics:
- Blend spinach or kale with frozen berries, banana, and kefir or yogurt.
- Pour into a bowl and top with granola, sliced fruits, and a drizzle of honey or nut butter.

3. Avocado Toast with Poached Egg:
- Spread mashed avocado on whole grain toast.
- Top with a poached egg, a sprinkle of salt and pepper, and a side of mixed greens for added fiber.

Gut-Healthy Breakfast Ideas

Gut-Healthy Breakfast Ideas

4. Chia Seed Pudding with Fruit:
- Mix chia seeds with milk (or a milk alternative) and let sit overnight in the refrigerator.
- In the morning, top with sliced fruits, such as mango or berries, and a handful of nuts or seeds.

5. Vegetable and Egg Breakfast Burrito:
- Fill a whole grain tortilla with scrambled eggs, sautéed spinach, bell peppers, and a sprinkle of cheese.
- Roll up and serve with salsa or avocado slices on the side.

Gut-Healthy Breakfast Ideas

Gut-Healthy Breakfast Ideas

Tips for Incorporating Gut-Healthy Breakfasts into Your Routine

Prepare Ahead: Many gut-healthy breakfast options can be prepared in advance or assembled quickly in the morning to accommodate busy schedules.

Experiment with Flavors: Add variety to your breakfast routine by experimenting with different fruits, vegetables, herbs, and spices to keep meals exciting and flavorful.

Hydrate: Pair your breakfast with a glass of water or herbal tea to support hydration and aid digestion.

Gut-Healthy Breakfast Ideas

Gut-Healthy Breakfast Ideas

Tips for Incorporating Gut-Healthy Breakfasts into Your Routine

Conclusion

By starting the day with nutrient-dense breakfast choices that prioritize gut health, mothers can nourish their bodies and set a positive tone for the day ahead. These gut-healthy breakfast ideas provide a delicious way to incorporate fiber, probiotics, and essential nutrients into your morning routine, supporting digestive health and overall well-being. In the subsequent chapters, we will explore lunch and dinner meal ideas designed to further enhance gut health and promote balanced nutrition for mothers and their families.

Chapter 7: Wholesome Lunch and Dinner Ideas

Lunch and dinner provide opportunities to nourish the body with balanced meals that support gut health and overall well-being. In this chapter, we explore wholesome lunch and dinner meal ideas designed for busy mothers looking to prioritize nutritious eating without sacrificing flavor or variety. These meal ideas incorporate ingredients that promote and support digestive health.

Wholesome Lunch and Dinner Ideas

Importance of Wholesome Meals

Lunch and dinner are significant meals that sustain energy levels and provide essential nutrients throughout the day. By focusing on wholesome ingredients and balanced meals, mothers can optimize their nutrition, support gut health, and foster a healthy relationship with food for themselves and their families.

Wholesome Lunch and Dinner Ideas

Key Components of Gut-Healthy Meals

1. Lean Proteins: Incorporate lean sources of protein such as poultry, fish, beans, lentils, tofu, or lean cuts of beef. Protein supports muscle repair, satiety, and overall health.

2. Fiber-Rich Vegetables: Include a variety of colorful vegetables such as leafy greens, broccoli, carrots, bell peppers, and zucchini.

Wholesome Lunch and Dinner Ideas

Key Components of Gut-Healthy Meals

3. **Whole Grains:** grains like brown rice, quinoa, whole wheat pasta, or barley. Whole grains are rich in fiber, B vitamins, and minerals that support digestive regularity and nourish beneficial gut bacteria.

4. **Healthy Fats:** Incorporate sources of healthy fats such as avocado, nuts, seeds, and olive oil. Healthy fats support gut lining integrity, reduce inflammation, and promote nutrient absorption.

Wholesome Lunch and Dinner Ideas

Wholesome Lunch and Dinner Meal Ideas

1. Grilled Chicken Salad with Quinoa:
- Grilled chicken breast served over a bed of mixed greens, quinoa, cherry tomatoes, cucumber, and avocado.
- Drizzle with a lemon-tahini dressing made with tahini, lemon juice, garlic, and olive oil.

2. Vegetarian Stir-Fry with Tofu:
- Stir-fry tofu cubes with colorful vegetables such as broccoli, bell peppers, snap peas, and carrots.
- Serve over brown rice or quinoa, seasoned with soy sauce, ginger, and garlic.

3. Salmon with Roasted Vegetables:
- Baked salmon fillets seasoned with herbs and served alongside roasted sweet potatoes, Brussels sprouts, and asparagus.
- Drizzle with a lemon-dill yogurt sauce made with Greek yogurt, lemon juice, dill, and garlic.

Wholesome Lunch and Dinner Ideas

Wholesome Lunch and Dinner Meal Ideas

4. Chickpea and Spinach Curry:

- Sauté onions, garlic, and spices like curry powder, turmeric, and cumin.
- Add chickpeas, diced tomatoes, and coconut milk, and simmer until flavors meld.
- Stir in fresh spinach just before serving and serve over brown rice.

5. Quinoa Stuffed Bell Peppers:

- Cook quinoa and mix with sautéed onions, garlic, black beans, corn, diced tomatoes, and spices.
- Stuff into halved bell peppers and bake until tender, garnish with fresh herbs.

Tips for Meal Preparation and Variety

Batch Cooking: Prepare components of meals in advance, such as cooking grains, chopping vegetables, or marinating proteins, to streamline meal preparation during busy weekdays.

Wholesome Lunch and Dinner Ideas

Wholesome Lunch and Dinner Meal Ideas

Experiment with Herbs and Spices: Use a variety of herbs, spices, and seasonings to add flavor without excess salt or unhealthy fats.

Include Fermented Foods: Fermented vegetables, such as sauerkraut or kimchi, to introduce probiotics that support gut diversity.

Wholesome Lunch and Dinner Ideas

Conclusion

Incorporating wholesome lunch and dinner ideas that prioritize lean proteins, fiber-rich vegetables, whole grains, and healthy fats will nourish your body and support gut health. These ideas offer a delicious and nutritious way to enjoy balanced meals that promote digestive health and overall well-being for mothers and their families. In the upcoming chapters, we will explore snacks, desserts, and lifestyle tips that enhance gut health and promote a holistic approach to wellness.

In the upcoming chapters, we will explore snacks, desserts, and lifestyle tips that further enhance gut health and promote a holistic approach to wellness.

Chapter 8: Snacks and Desserts for Gut Health

Snacking can be an opportunity to support gut health with nutrient-dense choices that satisfy cravings and provide energy between meals. In this chapter, we explore wholesome snack options and gut-friendly desserts designed to nourish mothers and promote a balanced approach to snacking.

Importance of Wholesome Snacking

Snacks play a important role in maintaining energy levels and preventing overeating during main meals. By choosing snacks that are rich in fiber, vitamins, minerals, and healthy fats, mothers can support gut health while satisfying hunger and cravings.

Snacks and Desserts for Gut Health

Components of Gut-Healthy Snacks

When selecting snacks that promote gut health, consider incorporating the following components:

1. Fiber-Rich Fruits and Vegetables: Choose fresh fruits and vegetables that are high in fiber, such as berries, apples, carrots, celery, and bell peppers.

2. Protein-Rich Options: Include snacks that provide protein to promote satiety and support muscle repair. Options include Greek yogurt, cottage cheese, nuts, seeds, and hummus.

Snacks and Desserts for Gut Health

Components of Gut-Healthy Snacks

3. Healthy Fats: Incorporate sources of healthy fats like avocado, nuts (such as almonds, walnuts), seeds (like chia seeds, flaxseeds), and olives.

4. Probiotic Foods: Introduce probiotics into snacks with options like yogurt with live cultures, kefir, or fermented vegetables (such as sauerkraut or kimchi).

Snacks and Desserts for Gut Health

Components of Gut-Healthy Snacks

Wholesome Snack Ideas

Here are some gut-healthy snack ideas to incorporate into your daily routine:

1. Greek Yogurt Parfait:
Layer Greek yogurt with fresh berries, a drizzle of honey, and a sprinkle of granola or crushed nuts for added crunch and fiber.

2. Vegetable Sticks with Hummus:
Enjoy crisp carrot, cucumber, and bell pepper sticks with a side of hummus for a satisfying snack packed with fiber and protein.

3. Chia Seed Pudding:
Mix chia seeds with almond milk and a touch of vanilla extract, let sit in the refrigerator until thickened.
Top with sliced fruits like mango or berries and a sprinkle of shredded coconut.

Snacks and Desserts for Gut Health

Components of Gut-Healthy Snacks

Wholesome Snack Ideas

4. Avocado Toast with Egg:

Spread mashed avocado on whole grain toast and top with a sliced hard-boiled egg, a dash of salt and pepper for a protein-packed snack.

5. Trail Mix:
Combine a mix of nuts (such as almonds, walnuts, and cashews), seeds (like pumpkin or sunflower seeds), and dried fruits (like apricots or raisins) for a portable and nutritious snack.

Gut-Friendly Desserts

Enjoying desserts can also align with gut health goals by choosing options that include wholesome ingredients and moderate sweetness:

Fruit and Yogurt Parfait: Layer Greek yogurt with sliced fruits like strawberries and kiwi, topped with a drizzle of honey or a sprinkle of dark chocolate chips.

Snacks and Desserts for Gut Health

Components of Gut-Healthy Snacks

Wholesome Snack Ideas

Homemade Fruit Sorbet: Blend frozen fruits like mango or berries with a splash of coconut water or almond milk until smooth and creamy.

Dark Chocolate Covered Almonds: Dip almonds in melted dark chocolate and let them cool on a parchment-lined tray for a satisfying sweet and crunchy treat.

Tips for Healthy Snacking

Portion Control: Enjoy snacks in moderation and practice mindful eating to avoid **overconsumption.**

Hydration: Pair snacks with water or herbal tea to support hydration and aid digestion.

Plan Ahead: Prepare snacks in advance and portion them into containers for easy grab-and-go options during busy days.

Snacks and Desserts for Gut Health

Conclusion

These snack and dessert ideas provide a balanced approach to snacking that promotes digestive health and overall well-being. In the following chapters, we will explore lifestyle tips and strategies that further enhance gut health and support mothers in their journey toward optimal wellness.

Chapter 9: Lifestyle Tips for Optimal Gut Health

Beyond diet, lifestyle choices play a significant role in supporting a healthy gut microbiome and overall well-being. This chapter explores practical lifestyle tips that mothers can incorporate into their daily routines to enhance gut health, manage stress, promote physical activity, and foster a balanced approach to wellness.

Managing Stress for Gut Health

Chronic stress can negatively impact gut health by altering the composition and function of the gut microbiome. Implementing stress management techniques can help mothers reduce stress levels and support digestive health:

Lifestyle Tips for Optimal Gut Health

Managing Stress for Gut Health

1. Mindfulness and Meditation: Practice mindfulness meditation or deep breathing exercises to promote relaxation and reduce stress hormones like cortisol.

2. Regular Exercise: Engage in regular physical activity such as yoga, walking, jogging, or dancing. Exercise helps regulate digestion, reduce inflammation, and support overall gut health.

3. Quality Sleep: Prioritize adequate sleep each night to support immune function, regulate appetite hormones, and promote overall well-being.

Lifestyle Tips for Optimal Gut Health

Hydration and Gut Health

Aim to drink at least 8-10 glasses of water daily, and increase intake during hot weather or physical activity to stay hydrated.

Lifestyle Tips for Optimal Gut Health

Avoiding Harmful Substances

Certain substances can disrupt gut health and contribute to digestive issues. Limiting or avoiding these substances can support a healthy gut microbiome:

1. **Limit Alcohol:** Consuming too much alcohol can disturb gut bacteria and hinder digestion. It's best to consume alcohol moderately, and you may want to consider alternatives such as herbal teas or infused water.

2. **Cut Back on Caffeine:** Consuming high amounts of caffeine can increase acid production in the stomach and impact gut motility. You may want to consider reducing your caffeine intake or choosing green tea, which contains antioxidants that promote gut health.

Lifestyle Tips for Optimal Gut Health

Regular Physical Activity

Incorporating regular physical activity into daily routines not only supports overall health but also promotes digestive regularity and gut microbiome diversity:

Aim for at least 30 minutes of moderate exercise most days of the week. Choose activities you enjoy, such as walking, cycling, swimming, or gardening.

Supporting Gut Health with Supplements

While a balanced diet is essential for gut health, some individuals may benefit from supplements to support digestive function and gut microbiome balance:

Lifestyle Tips for Optimal Gut Health

Supporting Gut Health with Supplement

Probiotic Supplements: Consider probiotic supplements containing strains beneficial for gut health. Consult with a healthcare provider to determine appropriate strains and dosage.

Digestive Enzymes: Digestive enzyme supplements can aid in the breakdown and absorption of nutrients, particularly for individuals with digestive disorders or deficiencies.

Practicing Good Hygiene and Food Safety

Maintaining good hygiene and food safety practices can help prevent infections and protect the gut microbiome:

Lifestyle Tips for Optimal Gut Health

Wash hands thoroughly before preparing or eating meals, and ensure proper storage and handling of food to prevent contamination.

Conclusion

From managing stress and staying hydrated to incorporating regular physical activity and practicing good hygiene, these practical strategies empower mothers to prioritize their health and nurture their families with a holistic approach to wellness. In the final chapter, we will summarize takeaways and provide a roadmap for continued success in maintaining optimal gut health for mothers and their loved ones.

Chapter 10: Summary and Roadmap to Optimal Gut Health

Throughout this ebook, we've explored essential strategies, meal plans, and lifestyle tips designed to empower mothers in supporting optimal gut health for themselves and their families. This final chapter summarizes key takeaways and provides a roadmap to continue fostering a healthy gut microbiome and overall well-being.

Recap of Key Concepts

1. Nutrient-Rich Diet: A diet rich in fiber, whole grains, lean proteins, healthy fats, probiotics, and prebiotics is fundamental for nurturing a diverse and balanced gut microbiome. These nutrients support digestion, immune function, and overall health.

2. Meal Planning: Planning meals in advance allows mothers to prioritize nutritious eating amidst busy schedules. By incorporating a variety of fruits, vegetables, proteins, and whole grains, mothers can create balanced meals that support gut health and provide essential nutrients.

Summary and Roadmap to Optimal Gut Health

Recap of Key Concepts

3. Gut-Healthy Meal Ideas: From breakfast ideas to wholesome lunch and dinner ideas, we've explored delicious and nutritious meal options that promote digestive health. These ideas emphasize fiber, probiotics, and nutrient-dense ingredients to support a thriving gut microbiome.

4. Snacks and Desserts: Incorporating snacks and desserts that prioritize fiber, protein, healthy fats, and probiotics provides additional opportunities to support gut health throughout the day. These wholesome options satisfy cravings while promoting digestive regularity and overall well-being.

5. Lifestyle Factors: Managing stress, staying hydrated, engaging in regular physical activity, and practicing good hygiene are essential lifestyle factors that contribute to a healthy gut microbiome. These habits support digestive function, reduce inflammation, and enhance overall health.

Summary and Roadmap to Optimal Gut Health

Roadmap to Continued Success

To maintain and further enhance gut health beyond this ebook, consider the following roadmap:

1. Assess Your Current Diet: Take inventory of your current eating habits and identify areas where you can incorporate more fiber-rich foods, probiotics, and nutrient-dense options.

2. Plan Meals Weekly: Continue meal planning to ensure balanced nutrition and simplify grocery shopping. Experiment with new recipes and ingredients to keep meals exciting and varied.

3. Prioritize Gut-Healthy Foods: Incorporate a variety of fruits, vegetables, whole grains, lean proteins, healthy fats, probiotics, and prebiotics into your daily meals and snacks.

Summary and Roadmap to Optimal Gut Health

Roadmap to Continued Success

4. Practice Mindful Eating: Pay attention to hunger and fullness cues, and eat slowly to aid digestion and prevent overeating. Mindful eating promotes enjoyment of food and supports digestive health.

5. Manage Stress: Implement stress management techniques such as meditation, yoga, or deep breathing exercises to reduce stress levels and support a healthy gut microbiome.

6. Stay Hydrated: Drink plenty of water throughout the day to maintain hydration, support digestion, and flush out toxins from the body.

Summary and Roadmap to Optimal Gut Health

Roadmap to Continued Success

7. Stay Active: Incorporate regular physical activity into your routine to promote digestive regularity, reduce inflammation, and support overall health.

8. Monitor and Adjust: Pay attention to how your body responds to different foods and lifestyle choices. Make adjustments as needed to optimize gut health and well-being.

Summary and Roadmap to Optimal Gut Health

Conclusion

By implementing the strategies and recommendations outlined in this ebook, you can take proactive steps toward fostering optimal gut health for themselves and their families. From nutrient-rich meal plans and wholesome meal ideas to lifestyle tips that support digestive function and overall well-being, each chapter has provided valuable insights and practical guidance. Embrace these principles as a foundation for a healthy lifestyle, and continue to prioritize gut health as a cornerstone of wellness. Please consult with your doctor before attempting any tips within this e-book. Here's to thriving health and vitality for you and your loved ones!

Bonus Chapter: Stretching for Gut Health

Stretching is often associated with improving flexibility and relieving muscle tension and its benefits extend beyond physical flexibility. In this bonus chapter, we explore how adding stretching exercises into your routine can support gut health and overall well-being.

Understanding the Gut-Brain Connection

The gut-brain axis is a bidirectional communication system between the gut and the brain, linking emotional and cognitive centers of the brain with peripheral intestinal functions. Stress and anxiety can impact this axis, leading to digestive discomfort and altered gut composition. Stretching can play a crucial role in reducing stress and promoting relaxation, thereby positively influencing gut health.

Bonus Chapter:
Stretching for Gut Health

Benefits of Stretching for Gut Health

1. Reduction of Stress and Anxiety: Stretching exercises promote relaxation by releasing tension in muscles and promoting blood flow.

2. Enhanced Digestive Function: Gentle stretches can stimulate the abdominal muscles and improve circulation to the digestive organs, promoting more efficient digestion and nutrient absorption.

3. Improved Posture: Maintaining good posture through stretching exercises can prevent digestive issues like acid reflux and bloating, as proper alignment supports optimal function of the gastrointestinal tract.

Bonus Chapter:
Stretching for Gut Health

4. Promotion of Mindfulness: Stretching encourages mindfulness by focusing on the body and breath. Mindful stretching sessions can reduce emotional eating, support healthy food choices, and enhance overall awareness of gut health.

Stretching Exercises for Gut Health

Incorporate these gentle stretching exercises into your daily routine to support gut health:

1. Child's Pose (Balasana):
- Kneel on the floor, sit back on your heels, and stretch your arms forward with your forehead resting on the mat or floor.
- Hold for 30 seconds to 1 minute, focusing on deep breathing to relax the body and mind.

2. Seated Forward Bend (Paschimottanasana):
- Sit on the floor with legs extended in front of you. Reach your arms toward your feet, keeping your spine long.
- Hold onto your feet or shins and gently fold forward from the hips.
- Hold for 30 seconds to 1 minute, breathing deeply to release tension in the lower back and promote digestion.

Bonus Chapter:
Stretching for Gut Health

Stretching Exercises for Gut Health

3. Twisting Seated Stretch:
- Sit cross-legged on the floor or in a chair with your spine tall.
- Place your left hand on your right knee and gently twist your torso to the right, placing your right hand behind you for support.
- Hold for 20-30 seconds, then repeat on the opposite side.
- Twisting stretches stimulate digestion and relieve bloating by massaging the internal organs.

Bonus Chapter:
Stretching for Gut Health

Stretching Exercises for Gut Health

4. Cat-Cow Stretch :
- Start on your hands and knees with your wrists aligned under your shoulders and knees under your hips.
- Inhale as you arch your back, dropping your belly towards the floor (Cow Pose).
- Exhale as you round your spine towards the ceiling, tucking your chin to your chest (Cat Pose).
- Repeat this flowing movement for 1-2 minutes, syncing breath with movement to massage the digestive organs and improve circulation.

5. Standing Side Stretch:
- Stand with your feet hip-width apart, arms by your sides.
- Reach your left arm overhead, bending gently to the right side.
- Hold for 20-30 seconds, feeling the stretch along the left side of your body.
- Repeat on the opposite side to stretch the abdominal muscles and promote relaxation.

Bonus Chapter:
Stretching for Gut Health

Stretching Exercises for Gut Health

5. Standing Side Stretch:
- Stand with your feet hip-width apart, arms by your sides.
- Reach your left arm overhead, bending gently to the right side.
- Hold for 20-30 seconds, feeling the stretch along the left side of your body.
- Repeat on the opposite side to stretch the abdominal muscles and promote relaxation.

Incorporating Stretching into Your Routine

Consistency: Aim to stretch daily or incorporate stretching into your warm-up or cool-down routines.
Mindfulness: Practice deep breathing and mindfulness during stretching exercises to enhance relaxation and stress reduction.

Bonus Chapter: Stretching for Gut Health

Incorporating Stretching into Your Routine

Variety: Explore different stretching techniques to target different muscle groups and promote overall flexibility and well-being.

Conclusion

By incorporating gentle stretching exercises into your daily routine, you can promote gut health by reducing stress, improving digestion, enhancing and promoting your overall well-being.Embrace these stretching techniques as part of a holistic approach to health, combining them with nutritious eating habits, regular physical activity, and stress management strategies. Strengthening the gut-brain connection through stretching can enhance your quality of life and contribute to a healthier, happier you.

A Healthier you :

Throughout this ebook, we've explored the intricate relationship between diet, lifestyle, and gut health, offering practical strategies and delicious meal ideas to empower mothers in fostering optimal well-being. A healthy gut is not just about digestion; it influences immunity, mood, and overall vitality. By prioritizing fiber-rich foods, probiotics, and mindful eating, mothers can nurture a diverse gut microbiome that supports digestive function and boosts immune resilience.

Beyond nutrition, incorporating stress management techniques, regular physical activity, and adequate hydration further enhances gut health. Each decision— from meal planning to stretching routines— contributes to a holistic approach to wellness. Remember, small changes add up to significant improvements over time.

As you embark on your journey to prioritize gut health, continue exploring new flavors, recipes, and self-care practices that resonate with your lifestyle. By nurturing your gut, you're nurturing your overall health and well-being, ensuring you have the energy and vitality to enjoy every moment with your loved ones. Here's to embracing a vibrant life fueled by a healthy gut!

www.ingramcontent.com/pod-product-compliance
Lightning Source LLC
Chambersburg PA
CBHW070802250726

48662CB00004B/1928